STRENGTH TRAINING FOR WOMEN OVER 60

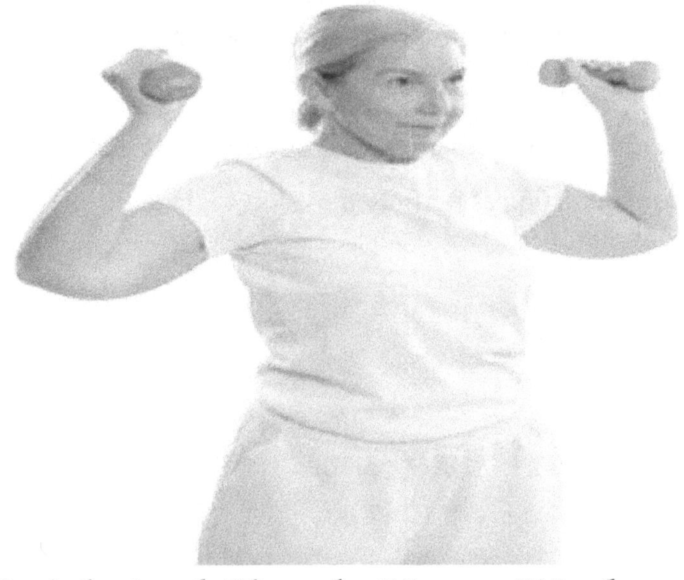

Quick And Simple Home Workouts For Beginners And Seniors To Build Muscles And Reclaim Energy, Balance And Mobility

Randy T. Lucas

Copyright 2024, Randy T. Lucas

Table of contents

INTRODUCTION

In a quiet corner of a bustling town, a group of extraordinary women, all over the age of 60, embarked on a remarkable journey that defied stereotypes and redefined what it means to age gracefully. Their story began with Evelyn, a lively 65-year-old who stumbled upon a revelation that would transform not just her life but the lives of her companions - the 'Strength Training for Women Over 60' guide.

Evelyn, seeking a spark to invigorate her routine, found herself captivated by this guide, brimming with tailored exercises specifically designed to suit the needs of mature women. Embracing it as her secret weapon, she embarked on a quest to reclaim her strength and vitality.

As the days turned into weeks, Evelyn's dedication and commitment bore fruit, evident not just in her physical prowess but in her infectious energy and unwavering confidence. Her friends, initially skeptical, witnessed her remarkable transformation. Mary, intrigued by Evelyn's newfound vigor, decided to join in, and soon discovered her own reservoir of strength. Sylvia, who believed age had dimmed her potential, found herself revitalized by the surge of energy she gained from these exercises.

Their weekly gatherings transformed from mere workouts into sessions filled with laughter, encouragement, and a shared sense of achievement. Each lifted weight symbolized more than just physical exertion; it signified their collective journey towards empowerment and renewed zest for life.

Through sweat and camaraderie, these women discovered a newfound resilience that transcended the confines of their workouts. Their muscles grew stronger, balance improved, and energy levels soared, but it was the newfound confidence and vitality that left an indelible mark on their lives.

Their transformative stories echoed beyond their close-knit circle, resonating with others in the community. More women, intrigued by the tales of renewed strength and invigoration, began seeking guidance from the 'Strength Training for Women Over 60' guide, sparking a movement of empowerment and liberation from age-related stereotypes.

Their journey serves as a testament to the transformative power of strength training, proving that age is not a barrier but a gateway to rediscovering one's strength and vitality. The 'Strength Training for Women Over 60' guide isn't just about lifting weights; it's about rewriting the narrative of aging, embracing resilience, and unlocking a vibrant and empowered chapter in one's life.

CHAPTER 1

Safety Tips and Precautions

1. Consult with a Healthcare Professional: Before beginning any new exercise program, especially strength training, consult with your healthcare provider to ensure it's safe for you and won't exacerbate any existing health conditions.

2. Learn Proper Technique: Proper form is crucial to prevent injuries. Consider hiring a certified personal trainer or joining a class to learn the correct techniques for exercises like squats, deadlifts, and bench presses.

3. Start Slowly and Progress Gradually: Begin with lighter weights and gradually increase the intensity as your strength improves. Rushing into heavy lifting can lead to strains or injuries.

4. Warm-Up and Cool Down: Always warm up your muscles with dynamic stretches or light cardio before starting your strength training routine. Similarly, end your session with static stretches to improve flexibility and prevent muscle soreness.

5. Use Appropriate Equipment: Ensure that the equipment you're using, such as weights, resistance bands, or machines, is suitable for your strength level and properly maintained to avoid accidents.

6. Listen to Your Body: Pay attention to your body's signals. If you experience pain, dizziness, or unusual discomfort during exercise, stop immediately and seek guidance from a fitness professional or healthcare provider.

7. Breathe Properly: Maintain a steady breathing pattern throughout your workouts. Exhale during the exertion phase (lifting, pushing, or pulling) and inhale during the relaxation phase.

8. Stay Hydrated: Drink water before, during, and after your strength training sessions to stay hydrated and maintain optimal performance. Dehydration can lead to fatigue and muscle cramps.

9. Rest and Recovery: Allow your muscles time to recover between sessions. Overtraining can lead to fatigue, decreased performance, and increased risk of injury. Aim for at least 48 hours of rest for each muscle group.

10. Use Spotter or Safety Measures: When attempting heavier lifts, especially with free weights, have a spotter or use safety equipment like a power rack or safety bars to prevent accidents or injuries in case you can't complete a rep.

Benefits Of Strength Training For Women

1. Increased Muscle Strength: Strength training helps build and maintain muscle mass, which naturally declines with age. This increase in strength aids in performing daily tasks, improving balance, and reducing the risk of falls.

2. Enhanced Bone Health: Weight-bearing exercises in strength training stimulate bone growth, reducing the risk of osteoporosis and fractures commonly associated with aging.

3. Improved Metabolism: Regular strength training helps boost metabolism, aiding in weight management by burning calories more efficiently and maintaining a healthy body composition.

4. Enhanced Joint Health: Strengthening muscles around the joints provides better support, reducing joint pain and improving overall joint function, which is particularly beneficial for individuals with arthritis.

5. Better Functional Ability: Strength training improves overall functional capacity, making everyday activities, like carrying groceries or climbing stairs, easier and more manageable.

6. Increased Energy Levels: Engaging in strength training can lead to increased energy and vitality, reducing feelings of fatigue and improving overall stamina and endurance.

7. Enhanced Mental Health: Exercise, including strength training, releases endorphins, promoting a positive mood, reducing stress, anxiety, and depression, and leading to improved mental well-being.

8. Improved Sleep Quality: Regular exercise, including strength training, contributes to better sleep patterns, resulting in more restful and rejuvenating sleep.

9. Management of Chronic Conditions: Strength training can help manage chronic conditions like diabetes, heart disease, and hypertension by improving cardiovascular health, blood sugar control, and overall fitness levels.

10. Increased Independence and Quality of Life: By improving strength, mobility, and overall health, strength training empowers women over 60 to maintain independence, enjoy an active lifestyle, and enhance their overall quality of life as they age.

Tools And Equipment Needed For This Exercise

1. Dumbbells: Essential for exercises like dumbbell bicep curls, seated dumbbell shoulder presses, and many others. They provide resistance for targeting various muscle groups and are available in different weights based on individual strength levels.

2. Resistance Bands: Used for seated leg presses, leg curls, lateral leg raises, and more. They offer resistance similar to weights but with the advantage of being portable, allowing for a range of resistance levels.

3. Stability Ball: Employed for exercises such as seated Russian twists, seated leg presses against the ball, or stability ball crunches. It provides an unstable surface, engaging core muscles for stability and strength.

4. Chair or Bench: Essential for chair squats, seated knee extensions, and tricep dips using a chair. These support exercises that require sitting or resting positions and are easily accessible in most households.

5. Medicine Ball or Dumbbell: Used for exercises like overhead tricep extensions, standing Russian twists, or woodchoppers. These weighted tools add resistance and challenge the core and upper body muscles.

6. Yoga Mat: Utilized for floor exercises like bridges, dead bugs, or planks. It provides a comfortable surface and prevents slipping during floor-based workouts.

7. Ankle Weights: Worn during standing or lying leg exercises such as standing leg raises, side leg raises, or seated leg extensions. They add resistance to strengthen lower body muscles.

WARM UP EXERCISES AND STRETCHES

1. Arm Circles:

- **Starting Position:** Stand with feet shoulder-width apart, arms extended to the sides at shoulder height.

- **Steps:** Begin by making small circles with your arms, gradually increasing the size of the circles. Continue for 15-20 repetitions in each direction (clockwise and counterclockwise).

- **Purpose:** Arm circles warm up the shoulder joints and muscles, improving flexibility and mobility in the upper body.

2. Leg Swings:

- Starting Position:

Stand near a wall or sturdy object for support. Hold onto the support with one hand while standing on the other leg.

- Steps:

Swing the free leg forward and backward, maintaining a straight leg, for 10-15 repetitions. Then switch to swing the leg side to side.

- Purpose:

Leg swings dynamically stretch the hip flexors, hamstrings, and groin muscles, improving hip mobility and flexibility.

3. Cat-Cow Stretch:

- Starting Position:

Begin on your hands and knees in a tabletop position, with wrists aligned under shoulders and knees under hips.

- Steps:

Inhale and arch your back, dropping your belly towards the floor (Cow position). Exhale and round your spine, tucking your chin to your chest (Cat position).
Repeat for 10-15 repetitions.

- Purpose:

This stretch mobilizes the spine, stretches the back muscles, and improves flexibility in the spine and neck.

4. Standing Quadriceps Stretch:

- Starting Position:

Stand tall, holding onto a chair or wall for balance if needed.

- Steps:

Bend one knee and bring your foot towards your glutes, grabbing your ankle or foot with the hand on the same side. Hold the stretch for 20-30 seconds. Switch legs and repeat.

- Purpose:

This stretch targets the quadriceps muscles in the front of the thigh, improving flexibility and reducing tension.

5. Shoulder Stretch with Arm Across Chest:

- Starting Position:

Stand tall, keeping your feet shoulder-width apart.

- Steps:

Bring one arm across your chest, holding it with your opposite hand at the elbow. Pull the arm closer to your body slowly, and hold the stretch for 20 to 30 seconds. Switch arms and repeat.

- Purpose:

This stretch loosens the shoulder and upper back muscles, improving flexibility and range of motion in the shoulder joint.

CHAPTER 2

EXERCISES

1. Bodyweight Squats:

- Starting Position:

Stand with feet shoulder-width apart, toes slightly pointed outward, and hands clasped in front of the chest.

- Steps:

Lower your body by bending your knees and hips, as if sitting back into an imaginary chair. Keep your back straight and chest lifted. Lower until thighs are parallel to the floor, then return to the starting position. Aim for 10-15 repetitions.

- Purpose:

Bodyweight squats strengthen the lower body, including the quadriceps, hamstrings, glutes, and improve functional movements like sitting and standing.

2. Standing Calf Raises:

- Starting Position:

Stand tall, holding onto a chair or wall for balance if needed, with feet hip-width apart.

- Steps:

Slowly rise onto the balls of your feet, lifting your heels as high as possible. Hold for a moment at the top, then lower your heels back down. Aim for 12-15 repetitions.

- Purpose:

This exercise targets the calf muscles, improving ankle stability and strength for better balance and mobility.

3. Seated Leg Press (Using Resistance Bands):

- Starting Position:

Sit on a chair with your back straight and a resistance band looped around the bottom of one foot. Anchor the other end of the band under the opposite foot.

- Steps:

Press the foot with the resistance band forward, extending your leg against the band's resistance, then slowly return to the starting position. Complete 10-12 repetitions on each leg.

- Purpose:

Seated leg presses strengthen the quadriceps and hamstrings, improving lower body strength and stability.

4. Bent-Over Dumbbell Rows:

- Starting Position:

Stand with feet hip-width apart, holding a dumbbell in each hand. Bend your knees slightly and hinge forward at the hips, keeping your back straight.

- Steps:

Pull the dumbbells towards your hips by bending your elbows, squeezing your shoulder blades together. Lower the weights back down with control.
Perform 10-12 repetitions.

- Purpose:

Bent-over rows target the upper back muscles, including the lats and rhomboids, improving posture and upper body strength.

5. Wall Push-Ups:

- Starting Position:

Stand facing a wall, about arm's length away. Place your palms on the wall at shoulder height and slightly wider than shoulder-width apart.

- Steps:

Lower your body towards the wall by bending your elbows, keeping your body in a straight line. Push back to the starting position.

Aim for 8-12 repetitions.

- Purpose:

Wall push-ups strengthen the chest, shoulders, and triceps, promoting upper body strength and toning.

6. Bridge Exercise:

- Starting Position:

Lie on your back with knees bent and feet flat on the floor, hip-width apart. Arms should be resting by your sides.

- Steps:

Lift your hips off the ground by pressing through your heels, engaging your glutes and core muscles. Hold the bridge position for a few seconds, then lower your hips back down. Aim for 12-15 repetitions.

- Purpose:

Bridges strengthen the glutes, lower back, and core muscles, aiding in lower body stability and posture.

7. Standing Leg Raises:

- Starting Position:

Stand tall, holding onto a chair or wall for balance if needed.

- Steps:

Lift one leg straight out to the side, keeping it as straight as possible without leaning. Hold briefly at the top, then lower your leg back down.
Complete 10-12 repetitions on each leg.

- Purpose:

Standing leg raises target the hip abductor muscles, enhancing hip stability and improving balance.

8. Dumbbell Bicep Curls:

- Starting Position:

Stand with feet shoulder-width apart, holding a dumbbell in each hand, arms extended by your sides, palms facing forward.

- Steps:

Curl the dumbbells towards your shoulders by bending your elbows, keeping your upper arms stationary. Slowly lower the weights back down.
Aim for 10-12 repetitions.

- Purpose:

Bicep curls strengthen the biceps and forearms, improving arm strength for everyday tasks.

9. Chair Squats:

- Starting Position:

Sit on the edge of a sturdy chair with feet flat on the floor, hip-width apart.

- Steps:

Stand up from the chair by pushing through your heels, then slowly lower yourself back down, almost touching the chair without fully sitting.

Aim for 12-15 repetitions.

- Purpose:

Chair squats work the lower body muscles, particularly the quadriceps, glutes, and hamstrings, aiding in functional movements like sitting and standing.

10. Plank:

- Starting Position:

Begin on the floor face down, resting on your forearms and toes, elbows directly below the shoulders.

- Steps:

Lift your body off the ground, forming a straight line from head to heels, engaging your core muscles. Hold the plank position for 20-30 seconds, gradually increasing the duration as you build strength.

- Purpose:

Planks strengthen the core muscles, including the abs, back, and shoulders, improving overall stability and posture.

11. Lateral Leg Raises:

- Starting Position:

Stand tall, holding onto a chair or wall for support if needed.

- Steps:

Lift one leg out to the side while keeping it straight. Hold briefly at the top, then lower your leg back down.
Aim for 10-12 repetitions on each leg.

- Purpose:

Lateral leg raises target the hip abductor muscles, aiding in hip stability and balance.

12. Tricep Dips Using a Chair:

- Starting Position:

Sit on the edge of a sturdy chair, gripping the front edge with hands, fingers facing forward. Slide your bottom off the chair with legs extended and heels on the floor.

- Steps:

Bend your elbows to lower your body, then straighten your arms to lift back up. Aim for 10-12 repetitions.

- Purpose:

Tricep dips strengthen the triceps and shoulders, enhancing arm strength and toning.

13. Seated Row (Using Resistance Bands):

- Starting Position:

Sit on a chair with legs extended, securing a resistance band around your feet and holding the ends in each hand.

- Steps:

Pull the resistance bands towards your torso, squeezing your shoulder blades together. Slowly release the bands back to the starting position. Aim for 10-12 repetitions.

- Purpose:

Seated rows target the upper back and biceps, improving posture and upper body strength.

14. Wall Sit:

- Starting Position:

Lean against a wall with your back flat against it, then slide down until your knees are bent at a 90-degree angle, thighs parallel to the floor.

- Steps:

Hold the position, keeping your back against the wall, for 20-30 seconds or longer as you build strength.

- Purpose:

Wall sits strengthen the quadriceps, hamstrings, and glutes, improving lower body endurance and stability.

15. Dead Bug Exercise:

- Starting Position:

Lie on your back with arms extended straight up toward the ceiling, legs bent at a 90-degree angle, knees stacked over hips.

- Steps:

Lower one arm and the opposite leg toward the floor without touching it, then return to the starting position. Alternate sides.

Aim for 10-12 repetitions on each side.

- Purpose:

The dead bug exercise strengthens the core muscles and improves stability and coordination.

16. Side Leg Lifts (Seated):

- Starting Position:

Sit tall in a chair with back straight and feet flat on the floor.

- Steps:

Lift one leg to the side, keeping it straight, then slowly lower it back down. Alternate legs and aim for 10-12 repetitions on each side.

- Purpose:

Side leg lifts target the hip abductor muscles, improving hip stability and strengthening the outer thighs.

17. Standing Heel Raises:

- Starting Position:

Stand with feet shoulder-width apart, arms by your sides.

- Steps:

Rise onto your tiptoes as high as you can, then slowly lower
your heels back down.
Aim for 12-15 repetitions.

- Purpose:

This exercise strengthens the calf muscles, enhancing ankle
stability and lower leg strength.

18. Seated Knee Extensions (Using Resistance Bands):

- Starting Position:

Sit in a chair with feet flat on the floor and loop a resistance band around one foot, securing the other end under the chair's leg.

- Steps:

Extend your leg straight out, stretching the resistance band, then slowly bend your knee to return to the starting position. Aim for 10-12 repetitions on each leg.

- Purpose:

Seated knee extensions target the quadriceps, improving knee strength and stability.

19. Hamstring Curls (Using Resistance Bands):

- Starting Position:

Sit on the edge of a chair with feet flat on the floor, loop a resistance band around one ankle, securing the other end under the chair.

- Steps:

Bend your knee and bring your heel towards your glutes, then slowly extend your leg back out.
Aim for 10-12 repetitions on each leg.

- Purpose:

Hamstring curls strengthen the hamstring muscles, aiding in knee stability and flexibility.

20. Shoulder Blade Squeeze:

- Starting Position:

Sit or stand tall with shoulders relaxed.

- Steps:

Squeeze your shoulder blades together as if trying to hold a pencil between them. Hold the squeeze for 5-10 seconds, then relax.

Aim for 10-12 repetitions.

- Purpose:

The shoulder blade squeeze exercise targets the upper back muscles, promoting better posture and reducing upper back tension.

21. Standing Hip Abduction:

- Starting Position:

Stand tall, holding onto a chair or wall for support if needed.

- Steps:

Lift one leg sideways away from your body, keeping it straight. Hold briefly, then lower the leg back down.
Aim for 10-12 repetitions on each leg.

- Purpose:

This exercise targets the hip abductor muscles, improving hip stability and strength.

22. Standing Knee Flexion (Using Resistance Bands):

- Starting Position:

Stand tall, loop a resistance band around one ankle, anchoring the other end to a sturdy object.

- Steps:

Bend your knee, bringing your heel towards your glutes against the resistance of the band, then slowly straighten your leg.

Aim for 10-12 repetitions on each leg.

- Purpose:

Standing knee flexion strengthens the hamstrings and aids in knee stability and mobility.

23. Seated Shoulder Press (Using Dumbbells or Resistance Bands):

- Starting Position:

Sit on a chair with back straight, holding dumbbells or resistance bands in each hand at shoulder height.

- Steps:

Press the weights overhead until arms are fully extended, then slowly lower them back down.
Aim for 10-12 repetitions.

- Purpose:

Seated shoulder presses target the deltoid muscles, improving shoulder strength and mobility.

24. Leg Adduction (Using Resistance Bands):

- Starting Position:

Sit on a chair with knees bent and a resistance band looped around both thighs just above the knees.

- Steps:

Squeeze your thighs together against the resistance of the band, then slowly release.
Aim for 12-15 repetitions.

- Purpose:

Leg adduction strengthens the inner thigh muscles, enhancing hip stability and strength.

25. Overhead Tricep Extension (Using Dumbbells or Resistance Bands):

- Starting Position:

Stand or sit with back straight, holding a dumbbell or resistance band with both hands overhead.

- Steps:

Lower the weight behind your head by bending your elbows, then extend your arms back up.

Aim for 10-12 repetitions.

- Purpose:

Overhead tricep extensions target the triceps, improving arm strength and tone.

26. Seated Leg Press (Using a Stability Ball):

- Starting Position:

Sit on a stability ball with feet flat on the floor and the ball against a wall for stability. Place a resistance band around the thighs, just above the knees.

- Steps:

Press your feet into the floor, extending your legs until almost straight, then return to the starting position.
Aim for 10-12 repetitions.

- Purpose:

Seated leg press using a stability ball targets the quadriceps, hamstrings, and glutes, promoting lower body strength and stability.

27. Side Leg Raises (Using a Resistance Band):

- Starting Position:

Attach a resistance band around both ankles while standing or lying on one side with legs straight and stacked.

- Steps:

Lift the top leg upward against the resistance band, then slowly lower it back down.

Aim for 10-12 repetitions on each side.

- Purpose:

This exercise focuses on the outer thigh muscles (abductors), enhancing hip stability and strength.

28. Seated Dumbbell Shoulder Shrugs:

- Starting Position:

Sit on a chair with back straight, holding dumbbells in each hand by your sides, palms facing inward.

- Steps:

Elevate your shoulders towards your ears in a shrugging motion, then lower them back down.
Aim for 12-15 repetitions.

- Purpose:

Seated shoulder shrugs target the upper trapezius muscles, aiding in shoulder strength and stability.

29. Standing Leg Curl (Using Resistance Bands):

- Starting Position:

Stand tall, loop a resistance band around one ankle, securing the other end to a sturdy object in front of you.

- Steps:

Bend your knee, pulling your heel towards your glutes against the resistance of the band, then slowly straighten your leg.

Aim for 10-12 repetitions on each leg.

- Purpose:

Standing leg curls strengthen the hamstring muscles and improve knee stability and flexibility.

30. Seated Russian Twists (Using a Medicine Ball or Dumbbell):

- Starting Position:

Sit on the floor with knees bent, holding a medicine ball or dumbbell with both hands close to the chest.

- Steps:

Lean back slightly and twist your torso to one side, touching the weight to the floor beside you, then twist to the other side.

Aim for 12-15 repetitions on each side.

- Purpose:

Seated Russian twists engage the core muscles, enhancing abdominal strength and stability.

CONCLUSION

Strength training for women over 60 is not just about lifting weights; it's a transformative journey that encompasses empowerment, health, and rejuvenation. As we age, the importance of maintaining strength, mobility, and independence becomes increasingly evident. Fortunately, embracing a regular strength training regimen offers a multitude of benefits that extend far beyond the physical realm.

Throughout this journey, women over 60 witness remarkable changes in their bodies and minds. Engaging in strength training fosters an environment where resilience thrives, muscles strengthen, and confidence blossoms. Improved muscle strength and bone density gained from these exercises are not merely about physical appearance but about enhancing daily functionality and reducing the risk of injuries or falls.

Moreover, the mental and emotional benefits are equally profound. Strength training serves as a source of empowerment, promoting a positive mindset, reducing stress, and enhancing overall well-being. The sense of accomplishment derived from surpassing personal fitness milestones contributes to a more fulfilling life.

By consistently integrating strength training into their lives, these women defy stereotypes and embrace the true potential of aging gracefully. They not only inspire others but also set a precedent for breaking barriers and exploring new capabilities, regardless of age.

To those embarking on this journey, remember this: each repetition, each session, and each effort you put into strength training is a testament to your resilience and determination. Let the progress you make be your motivation. Embrace the changes in your body, celebrate every milestone, and never underestimate the power you hold within. Your journey towards strength is a journey towards a healthier, more vibrant, and fulfilling life. Keep pushing forward, stay committed, and witness the remarkable transformations that await you, empowering you to live life to the fullest.

FITNESS

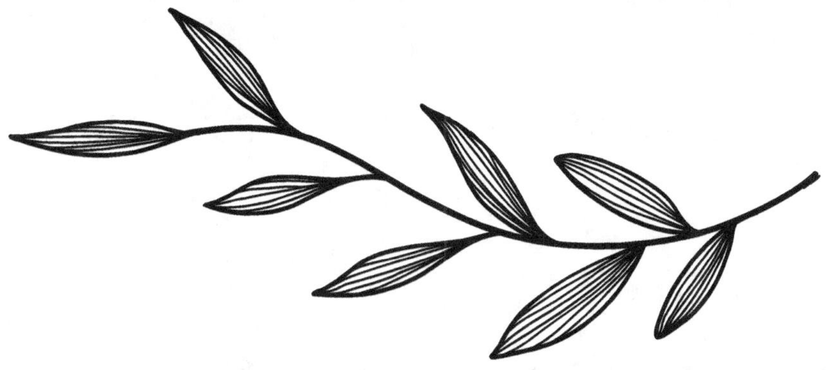

PLANNER

Fitness Planner

NAME:

DATE:

BREAKFAST

LUNCH

DINNER

SNACK

EXERCISE

SET

REP

NOTES

Fitness Planner

NAME: DATE:

BREAKFAST   LUNCH

DINNER   SNACK

EXERCISE   SET   REP   NOTES

Fitness Planner

NAME: **DATE:**

BREAKFAST

LUNCH

DINNER

SNACK

EXERCISE

SET	REP	NOTES

Fitness Planner

NAME: **DATE:**

BREAKFAST

LUNCH

DINNER

SNACK

EXERCISE

SET   REP   NOTES

Fitness Planner

NAME: **DATE:**

BREAKFAST

LUNCH

DINNER

SNACK

EXERCISE

SET	REP	NOTES

Fitness Planner

NAME: **DATE:**

BREAKFAST

LUNCH

DINNER

SNACK

EXERCISE

SET   REP   NOTES

Fitness Planner

NAME:　　　　　　　　　　**DATE:**

BREAKFAST

LUNCH

DINNER

SNACK

EXERCISE	SET	REP	NOTES

Fitness Planner

NAME: **DATE:**

BREAKFAST

LUNCH

DINNER

SNACK

EXERCISE

SET	REP	NOTES

Fitness Planner

NAME: **DATE:**

BREAKFAST

LUNCH

DINNER

SNACK

EXERCISE   SET   REP   NOTES

Fitness Planner

NAME: DATE:

BREAKFAST   **LUNCH**

DINNER   **SNACK**

EXERCISE   **SET**   **REP**   **NOTES**